AF285110

www.Insider-Heilverfahren.com
Hochwertig wissenschaftliche Gesundheitsliteratur

Die Werke des Medizinmann-Autors

Christian Meyer-Esch

Dear reader,

I am pleased that you have chosen my book.

Most people only know castor oil as a laxative.

But so far only known in insider circles is the fact that a dozen diseases have already been cured with the help of castor oil. Whether severe allergies, tinnitus, hair loss / balding, histamine intolerance, acne, migraines and even myopia and much more. All these healing successes are based on the experience of people who have tried it and whose experience reports have been written down in this book. In addition, the book provides specialist information about the exact mechanism of action and the prostaglandins, you will learn precise instructions for detoxification and everything you need to know about castor oil.

Environmental toxins such as heavy metals, pesticides and other chemical cocktails are on the rise, requiring efficient means of removing toxins from the body. With castor oil, nature has provided us with a gentle, safe and effective remedy whose detoxifying effects were previously only known in insider circles and are still known today.

At the back of the book you will find a castor oil log in which you can enter the detoxifications you have already completed. In this way you always have precise documentation of how many diversions you have already made and where you may have missed a diversion. Possible successes can also be entered there in the comment field.

Sincerely,

Her

Christian Meyer-Esch

Table of Contents ▼

Castor oil is obtained from the seeds of the castor, the so-called "miracle tree". The name says it all and really hits the nail on the head. Because all the miracles castor oil has done so far can hardly be understood by the human mind. Castor oil is obtained from the castor oil plant (Ricinus communis). She grows up extremely quickly. A height of five meters is reached after just a few months. The tallest plant is said to be thirteen

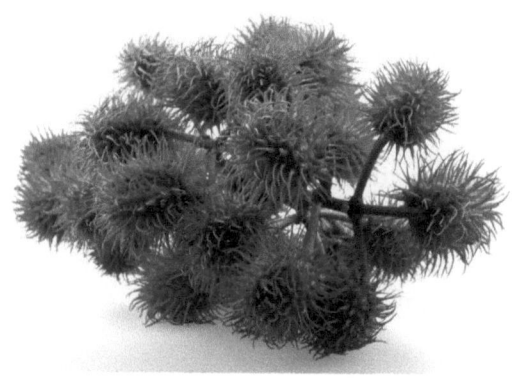

meters high. It prefers to grow in warm, sunny areas such as North Africa. Castor bean needs a lot of sun, but it also survives longer periods of drought. The oil is pressed from the highly toxic seeds of the plant, which contain the protein ricin. However, this toxic protein is no longer contained in the oil! Although castor oil has a strong laxative effect, it is absolutely harmless. It is translucent to yellowish in colour. You This sacred oil is truly not a new invention. This is one of the oldest natural remedies since human history. In the Middle Ages, castor oil was mainly used as a fuel for oil lamps and of course also for medicinal purposes. Nowadays, castor oil is mainly used in the cosmetics industry, in addition to its use as a laxative. E.g. as a shoe polish or as an additive for eyelashes and lips. And although the detoxifying effect of castor oil has been known for a long time, the healing knowledge has been forgotten. Castor oil has only experienced a renaissance in the past few years (at least in alternative medicine insider circles). In the mainstream, of course, the healing properties are unknown to this day. You can find more information in the chapter „The mechanism of action of castor oil".

Fatty Acid Profile Castor Oil:

Omega 3	Omega 6	Omega 9
Alpha Linolenic Acid 0.5%	Linoleic acid 5%	Ricinoleic acid 90%
		Oleic acid 4%

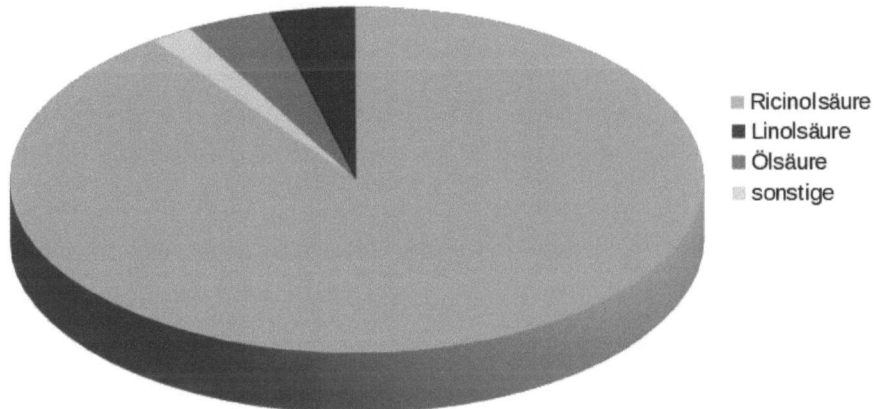

Ricinolsäure
Linolsäure
Ölsäure
sonstige

Toxic substances (toxins) are the cause of almost all diseases. Whether allergies, skin diseases or cancer. It cannot be overlooked that almost every disease is due to poisoning. In most cases, however, we are not acutely threatened by a toxin, but they enter the organism chronically, over a period of years. The following examples show how important regular detoxification is. We can hardly avoid all these sources of poison, because they are omnipresent. However, what we can do is detox regularly so that heavy metals, pesticides and other toxins have no place in our bodies. The increasing environmental pollution in western industrialized countries makes regular detoxification essential. The following examples are just a small excerpt from an unimaginable number of poison sources.

Cadmium in grain

Masses of cadmium are stored on agricultural soils. Wheat, rye and rice are particularly contaminated. Cadmium accumulates in the outer layers of the grain in particular, which is why the content in wheat bran is particularly high. The cadmium content in rye, barley and oats is slightly lower. Cadmium poisoning is associated with an increased risk of cancer and osteoporosis and also with kidney damage (studies 6, 7).

Lead in tap water

There are legally prescribed limit values for heavy metals in tap water. However, the waterworks are only obliged to ensure compliance with the limit values up to the end of their distribution network. Up until the mid-1970s, lead water pipes were often laid in Germany. Even today there are numerous buildings with lead pipes, which accumulate in the drinking water. Lead accumulation results in various deleterious effects on the central nervous system, primarily through increased oxidative stress (Study 8). 90% of lead accumulates in bones and teeth.

Lead and cadmium in cocoa and chocolate

One study examined the average lead concentration in cocoa beans. This was ≤ 0.5 ng/g, which is one of the lowest values for a natural food. In contrast, the lead concentrations of the manufactured cocoa and chocolate products were extremely high at 230 and 70 ng/g, respectively. A source of contamination of the finished products is tentatively attributed to atmospheric emissions from leaded gasoline still used in Nigeria (Study 9). Lead accumulation results in various deleterious effects on the central nervous system, primarily through increased oxidative stress (Study 8). 90% of lead accumulates in bones and teeth. Many cocoa varieties also come from cultivation areas in Latin America whose soils naturally have high levels of cadmium. This toxic metal is absorbed by the plant and thus ends up in the fruit. Some cocoa varieties therefore also contain increased cadmium levels.

Mercury in Fish & Seafood

Seas and rivers have a relatively high level of mercury contamination (depending on the pollution with sewage). Fish and seafood such as mussels are considered contaminated foods. The amount depends on the age and species of the fish and the degree of pollution in the water. However, fish that have been bred in aquaculture also have increased heavy metal values, since their animal feed is often contaminated with mercury. Tuna in particular is usually highly contaminated.

Lots of heavy metals in wild mushrooms

Heavy metals such as mercury or cadmium, which are blown out of exhaust pipes and industrial plants, end up in the ground via the air. Hardly any food is likely to be more heavily contaminated with heavy metals than mushrooms. Due to their fine structure, they store heavy metals and absorb them from the ground like a sponge. Mushrooms are real filters for the forest floor. For example, high cadmium levels have been found in some types of mushrooms and birch mushrooms in recent years. Lead was highly concentrated in porcini mushrooms, meadow mushrooms and chestnut boletes. Porcini mushrooms and aniseed mushrooms absorbed large amounts of mercury. Therefore, only buy cultivated organic mushrooms and no wild mushrooms!

On the following pages you will find reports on the various diseases. The experience reports were not taken over 1:1 with copy + paste, but interpreted and reproduced by me in terms of content. Of course, as always, no promises of healing are made! Just because castor oil has worked very well for others doesn't mean it has to work for you. But of course we hope that it will be the case with you too...

2 field reorts:
Chronic diarrhea and other gastrointestinal disorders

A patient who had been suffering from chronic diarrhea for 24 years (!) (cause apparently unclear) tested castor oil for the first time for purging and detoxification. Everything went smoothly. Only his bottom got a little sore. Already after the 1st discharge he had no more diarrhea 3 days later. And that after 24 years! He reported that he only had diarrhea once in that month. (Source: 1a)

A woman reports that after a few castor oil discharges, her gastrointestinal problems became less (Source 1b).

1 field report: Eczema

Here, a man reports that he got rid of the chronic itchy skin on the back of his hands after just 2 weeks by using castor oil topically. As he describes, his skin symptoms (eczema) have flared up latently and occasionally extremely for about 2-3 years. He rubbed his hands with castor oil every night for 2 weeks. (Source: 2a)

3 field reports: Tinnitus

A woman reports no more tinnitus after taking castor oil. According to her statements, it was the most effective and gentlest elimination. Even if they don't remember it so well for a few days afterwards, it was unlike algae and co. makeable. As part of the administration, they developed foul-smelling stools with burning bile. (Source3a)

Another woman reports that she often had tinnitus before the cleansing with castor oil. Sometimes right, sometimes left and since the castor oil detox this whistling has completely disappeared. (Source3b)

A man had been suffering from chronic tinnitus for some time. After a few instructions (number unknown), it disappeared completely for about 5 days after the respective discharge (Source3c).

Author's Note: This is a typical sign of intoxication. After a discharge, the organism is initially free of toxins (at least in the blood), but gradually more toxins move in and the symptoms appear again. Until the organism is completely free of toxins at some point. But the exact opposite can also often be observed, namely that a so-called "initial aggravation" occurs. Everyone reacts differently here. A prostaglandin deficiency is also possible. Since castor oil is a partial prostaglandin E2 analogue and 2 of the 4 prostaglandin receptors are occupied, which have a strong circulatory effect and tinnitus is usually a symptom of circulatory disorders, this would not be possible.

2 field reports: Allergies

A man who has been taking castor oil for about 20 years reports that after 7 years and 225 castor oil discharges he was able to cure a severe form of light/sun allergy. He also reports that he no longer needs sunglasses, even though he lives 750 meters above sea level. He also reports that the following symptoms have completely disappeared after detoxing with castor oil:

Fatigue, depression, mood lability, anxiety, agitation, poor memory, headache and body aches, increased salivation, stomatitis (inflammation of the lining of the mouth), gingivitis (inflammation of the gums), gastroenteritis (inflammation of the lining of the stomach and small intestine) and muscle twitching. According to his own statements, he has been draining weekly with castor oil for 20 years. (Source 4a)

Another castor oil user reports that after 1.5 years and weekly castor oil cleansing, he no longer has any allergies. (Source 4b)

3 field reports: Rosier, firmer skin

One woman reports that after detoxifying with castor oil for a few months, the skin on her face became much rosier and silkier, and people around her started asking her about it. (Source 5a)

And one man reports that his skin has tightened since the castor oil detox. (Source 5b)

Another man reports that he could cry with happiness after various castor oil detoxifications: his complexion has improved, the wrinkles around his eyes have smoothed out, the intraocular pressure has normalized, the muscle pain is gone and his vision is clearer. (Source: 5c)

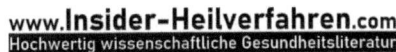

4 field reports: Hair loss and (male) pattern baldness

A woman reports that after a few months of taking castor oil, her scalp hair became significantly fuller and new hair also grew back in areas that were already bald. Her hair also grew back thicker. (Source 6a)

A man also reports that after some castor oil cleansing, his wife noticed that the hair on his head was growing again after it had been thinning for many years. Even with daily brushing, he noticed that there was hardly any hair loss. (Source 6b)

A castor oil user reports that he has suffered from hair loss for years. The hair on his head became thinner and thinner over the years. He's tried all kinds of remedies with no success. Recently he was even forced to only wash his hair with baby shampoo. After detoxing with castor oil for two months (9 drainages), he found that not only did his hair loss stop, but new hair started to grow in his receding hairline (source 6c).

Another castor oil user with a hand-sized bald spot on his head found that since the castor oil detoxes, something "more" than just fluff has been growing there again. He also found that external use in combination with sweating (e.g. sauna) brought a real growth boost (source 6d).

Note from the author: Since castor oil also stimulates hair growth when applied externally, it cannot be assumed that this has a detoxifying effect! Rather, castor oil will occupy the prostaglandin receptors EP3 and EP4 (Study 5). These then stimulate hair growth, similar to prostaglandin E2. So if you intend to use castor oil to stimulate hair growth, you are advised to take castor oil every day and in small doses (one teaspoon in the morning and one in the evening). Thus, the prostaglandin receptors are occupied around the clock and hair growth is stimulated. In this small dosage, castor oil usually does not have a laxative effect. And if you do, you can reduce the dose even further. Note, however, that castor oil taken orally stimulates hair growth all over the body and not just locally on the scalp. If hair growth is only desired on the scalp, you should combine the castor oil with DMSO so that the castor oil also reaches the deep layers of the skin. DMSO is a penetrant, i.e. an agent that promotes penetration into the skin and consists of sulfur. You can get DMSO in well-stocked online shops. But make sure that the environment is clean, as the DMSO also transports unwanted substances into the skin! For example, do not use plastic!

5 field reports: Acne and impure skin

One man reports that since the castor oil detox his skin has changed, becoming increasingly tight and free of any impurities (Source 7a)

One woman reports noticing clearer skin after 4 castor oil cleanses. (source 7b)

A woman who has had 16 castor oil discharges so far reports that she has hardly had any pimples on her upper arm since then (source 7c).

One woman reports that pimples, boils, and other "rough spots" on the skin go away right after a castor oil day (source 7d).

A castor oil user reports that since various discharges (he does not know the exact number), he has noticed "optically better skin". (source 7e)

2 field reports: short-sightedness (Myopia)

After completing 4 castor oil cleansings, a woman thought she was crazy when she suddenly realized her eyes were enlarging and she could suddenly see better with the short-sighted eye (source 8a).

After reading the above testimonial, a man confirmed his own experience of using castor oil for myopia. He used to be short-sighted on both sides with the values -2.5/-2.25, after massive poisoning with castor oil now only -1.0/-1.0 on both sides. Since then, he has only needed glasses when driving, especially at night (source 8b).

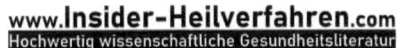

Author's Note: In my view, it is unlikely that the toxin drainage was the cause of the better vision in this case. It seems much more likely to me than if the mechanism of action was due to the promotion of prostaglandins. This would also explain why the freedom from symptoms often only lasted for a short time. So if you also suffer from myopia, try taking castor oil in small doses every day: one teaspoon in the morning and one teaspoon in the evening. I've tested this myself. I'm not short-sighted, but this small amount didn't have a laxative effect! If you also combine the castor oil with evening primrose oil, you also supply the linoleic acid and gamma-linolenic acid required for prostaglandin production. Castor oil occupies 2 out of 4 prostaglandin receptors, namely EP3 and EP4. The body needs the finished prostaglandins E1, E2 and E3 to occupy the receptors EP1 and EP2 (but of course also for EP3 and EP4). You can create these in your body with the oil combination
Borage oil or evening primrose oil + fish oil or
Borage oil or evening primrose oil + linseed oil.

3 field reports: Chronic fatigue

A woman reports that since the castor oil detox she is no longer constantly tired and therefore no longer has to lie down at midday (source 9a).

Another patient reports hardly ever being chronically tired after a 5-month, weekly castor oil detox. Furthermore, she is now much more concentrated and can follow conversations more attentively (source 9b).

Another castor oil user reports that she is no longer chronically tired after the 3rd drainage. Usually on Fridays, after a hard week's work, she was totally exhausted. But this time she was able to "uproot trees". She said she hadn't felt this energetic in decades(!) (source 9c).
A woman reports that she needs less sleep after various castor oil drainages. And she emphasized that she was very annoyed by the constant tiredness (source 9d).

1 field report: Back pain

A castor oil user reports that her back pain (sciatica) is gone except on days when she has her period or right after a castor oil day.
(Source 10a)

2 field reports: Histamine intolerance

A woman with histamine intolerance reports that her histamine intolerance improved significantly after just one drain. She ate a plaited nut and the sneezing and itching of the palate (which had otherwise occurred in the past) did not occur. The only side effect was very severe fatigue (source 11a).

Author's Note: Since chronic fatigue is usually greatly improved by castor oil, this is likely an initial aggravation. Something like this is quite common in detoxification cures.

A chronically ill patient with multiple symptoms reports that after 5 months of detoxing with castor oil at weekly intervals, she is now almost completely cured of histamine intolerance. Only with dishes that are extremely histamine-rich does she still get very few symptoms (source 11b).

1 field report: electro-sensitivity

A woman has been taking castor oil for 1.5 years, with a total of 29 discharges to date. Her symptoms prior to the start of the castor oil cleansing included severe electrical sensitivity, particularly sensitivity to cell phone radiation. She had headaches and dizziness at the time. Her experiences with castor oil were such that the symptoms worsened immediately after the cleansing (up to 1 week). Gradually, however, all symptoms subsided and the patient is now largely cured of electro-sensitivity (source 12a).

1 field report: Extreme sweating
A chronically ill woman who previously broke out in sweats regularly (triggered by minor exertion or vegetatively) has been taking castor oil for 5 months so far. Since then, the sweats have not only gotten better, they have completely disappeared. (Source 13a)

1 field report: pain in the musculoskeletal system
The same woman from the above experience report could hardly move her arms (e.g. when washing her hair) without pain. Since the 5-month detox with castor oil, she no longer has these problems (source 14a).

3 field reports: Migraines/Headaches
The same woman from the above experience report also suffered from chronic migraines and therefore needed strong painkillers. Since the 5-month detox with castor oil, the migraines have gotten significantly better. It hardly ever occurs and if it does, it is so slight that the patient no longer needs medication. (Source 15a)

Another woman reports that headaches disappear completely after a castor oil cleanse (source 15b)

A man reports that he no longer has a headache after being discharged several times (number unknown). (Source 15c)

One patient complained of headaches throughout the week. After detoxing with castor oil, the headache was gone the next day. (Source 15d)

1 field report: Various intolerances

A woman plagued by intolerances (lactose and most likely histamine) started the detox with castor oil. Since then she has had no more intolerances. Noodles with vanilla sauce or yeast dough are no longer a problem. Previously, she had asthmatic breathing problems and bloated stomach. Since the castor oil cleansing, she has been able to consume all of this again without any symptoms (source 16a).

1 field report: Cold and flu

One woman confirms that when she catches a cold, she hardly notices the cold after just one castor oil cleanse (source 17a).

1 field report: Elevated cadmium levels

A woman had a hair mineral analysis done before starting the castor oil detox. (Author's note: The body sends toxic metals such as cadmium into the scalp so that they can be removed from the body through the hair). The woman did a total of 33 castor oil discharges that year. In addition, she took chlorella algae and vitamins. The renewed hair mineral analysis showed that the cadmium value had dropped significantly. The woman did not reveal exact dates (18a).

1 field report: sleep disorders

A patient with insomnia reports that for the first time in 4 years he has been able to sleep 7 hours straight since the second castor oil drainage. Previously this was only possible for 3-4 hours (source 19a).

1 field report: pulling in the ear

A patient with chronic ear irritation (daily) noticed after the first castor oil drainage that 95% of it disappeared. Even 4 weeks later he had no more problems with it. He himself described this in his own words as a "miracle" (Source 20a).

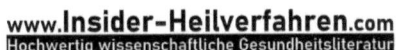

1 field report: numbness after heavy work
Here, a castor oil user reports that for many years after hard work (shoveling snow, carrying heavy things...) he has had numbness in his arms and legs at night. After a few castor oil discharges, these have now completely disappeared (21a).

1 field report: psoriasis/psoriasis
A man reports that he has had no more psoriasis since the weekly castor oil cleansing for 1.5 years (source 22a).

Precautions / Side Effects

• Purging with castor oil is only possible if the fat digestion is intact (gallbladder, pancreas). If there are gallstones, for example, taking castor oil is not recommended. Likewise not with problems of the pancreas. Gallstones and/or gallstones can usually be dissolved very well with 50 g of lecithin granules a day. However, lecithin itself is very high in fat. So if you have big problems with fat digestion, you should try choline + inositol in its pure form. Both can be bought cheaply as a powder in well-stocked internet shops.

• Since the laxative effect after taking castor oil occurs through the activation of histamines passively present in the small intestine, this is blocked by taking antihistamines. These must not be taken at the same time as taking castor oil and not two days before! Ask your doctor or pharmacist about the half-life (the time it takes for the active ingredient to break down) of the drug in question. There are also some anti-histamines in nature, such as oregano oil or thyme oil. These remedies block diarrhea! Therefore, castor oil can no longer work and can lead to abdominal cramps!

• Castor oil should not be used during pregnancy, if there is an intestinal obstruction or if there is unclear abdominal pain.

• In very rare cases, castor oil intolerance occurs. This can possibly be remedied by taking a hawthorn berry supplement.

Do not detox with castor oil if you...
• Taking antihistamines (or stopping them 2 days before)
• are pregnant
• have gallstones / your fat digestion is disturbed
• have a blockage in your intestines or unexplained abdominal pain

---

Questions and Answers (Q&A)

Does castor oil cause allergies?

Since allergies have already been cured with castor oil, the opposite is likely to be the case. Throughout my research, I didn't find a single case of ingestion of castor oil leading to an allergy. Some believe that an allergy to castor oil cannot occur simply because ricinoleic acid is not metabolized in the body. From my point of view, however, the ricinoleic acid is metabolized very well. How else could the prostaglandin E2 effects be explained? For example, some have noticed increased hair growth through regular intake of castor oil. How should the ricinoleic acid get to the scalp if it cannot be metabolized at all? Therefore, from my point of view, a clear YES to the metabolism of ricinoleic acid and a very likely NO to triggering allergies.

Some pharmacists warn against castor oil, especially for detoxification, because they believe castor oil increases the absorption of toxins in the body. What do you think of it?

What is meant is that castor oil as an oil can improve the absorption of fat-soluble toxins. This problem should no longer exist if medicinal charcoal and/or chlorella algae are taken at the same time, as these bind the toxins in the intestine and cause them to be excreted.

Will I lose or gain weight with castor oil?

Usually, castor oil has no effect on body weight.

**I had my gallbladder removed.
Can I still detox with castor oil?**

There are already testimonials from people who have had their gallbladder removed. All reported problem-free discharge with castor oil. Accordingly, the application seems to work even if the gallbladder is no longer present. All information as always without guarantee and at your own risk!

Does castor oil also dissolve or drain gallstones?

Usually not. However, according to empirical medicine, lecithin granules could be an excellent means of dissolving them. 50 g a day have proven effective for this. Available as soy or sunflower lecithin at drugstores.

Can you detox with castor oil several times a week?

From my personal experience I can say that this is easily possible. However, the question is whether you have the time and can tolerate it. If you already have a sore baboon butt from detoxification, you should take things a little slower and only detoxify 1-2 times a week. Ultimately, everyone does well to listen to their own body feeling. If you're feeling good and you have time, why not every day? The faster the toxins leave the body, the better. Don't waste time. However, with every castor oil detox, you also lose a lot of fluid and minerals, especially potassium. You should fill this up the following day. E.g. with an ORGANIC banana juice (rich in potassium).

Is there any scientific evidence that castor oil actually detoxifies?

no Detoxification with castor oil is based purely on empirical medicine without any scientific evidence. However, the numerous reports of experience cannot be dismissed out of hand: whoever heals is right. However, scientific evidence for heavy metal elimination is available for other healing methods, which I also describe in more detail in this book (see: Other insider healing methods for detoxification).

Is castor oil also suitable as a remedy for acute poisoning?

In the case of acute poisoning, medicinal charcoal is the first choice. In addition to support, castor oil is of course also recommended in order to be able to drain the toxic bile. If the acute poisoning has lasted longer than 1 week, caution should be exercised with castor oil, as this could irritate the intestines too much. In such a case, it is better to only use the medicinal charcoal alone.

Since taking castor oil, my symptoms have worsened significantly. How is that to be rated?

Such so-called "initial aggravations" are quite normal. The field reports clearly showed that this is only a short-term initial aggravation, which then improves or disappears with ongoing detoxification. As with any detoxification, a large number of toxins are mobilized and excreted, so that the level of toxins in the blood can be increased for a short time. Therefore, it is important to combine castor oil with medicinal charcoal or do enemas.

What do you do when you're so disgusted by castor oil that you're throwing up on it?

If all else fails, just get castor oil in capsule form. These are available under the name "laxative capsules" in every drugstore. But make sure that it is actually castor oil and not another active ingredient.

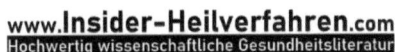

Where is the cheapest place to buy castor oil?

The 1 liter bottle is always the cheapest. Available in numerous online shops and pharmacies.

Can you eat before or after taking castor oil?
And if so, what and how much?

Everyone reacts differently here. I myself can fill my stomach before taking castor oil without any problems. However, I then only eat light food such as bread, chocolate or the like. In any case, you should avoid eating too greasy food. Because the more fat you eat, the more bile is released and this is then missing when the castor oil is metabolized. As a result, vomiting may occur. So refrain from excessive fat consumption, at least on castor oil day! Even after taking castor oil, I don't see any problems eating anything.

Science has already identified three mechanisms of action:

Mechanism of action 1: The occupation of 2 of 4 prostaglandin E receptors:

Castor oil or the ricinoleic acid it contains has a partially analogous effect to prostaglandin E2. This is a tissue hormone that the body produces itself from linoleic acid/arachidonic acid. The prostaglandin E2 occupies all 4 existing EP receptors from EP1 to EP4. Ricinoleic acid, on the other hand, only occupies 2 of these receptors, namely EP3 + EP4 (Study 5). Thus, castor oil is a partial prostaglandin E2 agonist. Occupying the EP3 and EP4 receptors primarily causes hair growth and the initiation of labor during pregnancy. Experience reports confirm that the regular intake of castor oil increased hair growth all over the body. This also affects men with so-called "hereditary" baldness. However, don't expect miracles here. Unfortunately, just because it encourages hair growth doesn't mean it will grow a lion's mane.

A number of diseases improved in studies treated with prostaglandins. So a deficit seems more than likely:

Disease:	Missing prostaglandin:
Poor hair growth, sparse eyebrows and eyelashes	E1, E2, F2-alpha
Glaucoma (increased pressure in the eye)	F2-alpha
Circulatory disorders	E1, E2, I2
Thrombosis	I2
Initiation of childbirth	E2
Grey hair	E2, F2a
Trigeminal neuralgia	E1
Autoimmune diseases	E1, Thromboxan A2
Cancer	E1, A1
Acne	E1
Premenstrual syndrome	E1

Mechanism of action 2: The drainage of the bile with interruption of the enterohepatic circulation:

The bile is a liquid stored in the gallbladder, which contains both fat-soluble toxic substances and is of crucial importance for the digestion of fat. It is therefore important to drain the bile as often as possible so that new bile can be produced. Because with every new production of bile, it is loaded with toxins from the whole body. Or to put it more comprehensibly: With every new production of bile, the body searches for toxins in all possible body tissues and deposits them in the bile so that from here a final elimination via the intestine is possible. At least that's the theory. That is not scientifically proven. However, it has been scientifically proven that toxins are stored in the bile. This can be looked up in any textbook. However, based on the numerous reports of experience with castor oil, it can be assumed that this is exactly the mechanism of action. Because the improvement of the symptoms only happens in the rarest of cases through a single discharge. Rather, it is the case that several drainages are needed and these can also be accompanied by initial aggravations. With each high-fat meal, bile is secreted into the duodenum. However, there is a catch: This only happens up to a maximum of 10%! The majority, i.e. 90%, is reabsorbed, i.e. recycled, so to speak, and migrates back to the gallbladder. This is called enterohepatic circulation (entero = intestine, hepatic = liver), i.e. "intestinal-liver circulation". Only castor oil causes 100% elimination of bile and thus also of toxins! On the one hand, castor oil is an oil (it stimulates the release of bile) and, on the other hand, it is also an agent that breaks the enterohepatic cycle. Therefore, castor oil cannot be compared to other laxatives such as Epsom salts. Because Epsom salt is not an oil and therefore cannot release bile.

Mechanism of action 3: New lymph vessels thanks to castor oil!

The lymphatic pathways in the body are our "sewage channels" through which the body detoxifies. The more lymphatic vessels there are in the body, the better the detoxification works. According to a study (10) from 2011, agents that stimulate the prostaglandin receptors EP3 and EP4 (which is the case with castor oil) cause the formation of new lymphatic vessels. This could explain why castor oil applied topically works for many. If you want to form new lymphatic vessels with the help of castor oil, it is also advisable to take it in small doses, such as 1 teaspoon twice a day, in addition to the weekly detoxification. In this small amount, castor oil usually has no laxative effect. If you do, you can block the diarrhea with a few drops of thyme oil or oregano oil. Since these essential oils block histamine and the laxative effect of castor oil works via histamine, castor oil does not cause diarrhea. You should therefore not take any antihistamines such as thyme oil / oregano oil on the detox day or two days before!

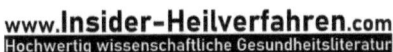

The human body produces up to 700 ml of bile every day, which is stored in the gallbladder. Bile is produced in the liver by hepatocytes (liver cells). The bile consists for the most part (approx. 80%) of water in which numerous substances are dissolved. These include lecithin, cholesterol, conjugated bile salts, hormones and bilirubin (the breakdown product of the red blood pigment hemoglobin). And what is particularly interesting for us: Medicines (residues), heavy metals, pesticides and other toxins that have no place in the human body and are just waiting to be finally excreted are also sent into the bile. Many substances stored in the bile are conjugated with glutathione (made water-soluble) and are thus more or less parked in the bile. The bile is thickened to about ten percent of its volume. If lipids (fats) get into the small intestine with food, they produce the hormone cholecystokinin (CCK) in the small intestinal mucosa. CCK stimulates the smooth muscle in the wall of the gallbladder to contract and mix its contents with the chyme in the duodenum. So whenever we ingest a fat from food, the bile is secreted from the gallbladder into the duodenum. On the one hand, it serves to digest fat, but on the other hand it also neutralizes the acidic chyme coming out of the stomach. Unfortunately, there is also the so-called "enterohepatic circulation". This causes only about 10% of the bile to leave the body through the bowel movements. The remaining 90% are reabsorbed, so to speak recycled. In a toxin-free body, this function may be useful to save bile. In a poisoned organism, on the other hand, this is fatal. And this is exactly where castor oil comes into play: This causes the enterohepatic circulation to be broken and thus all the bile can leave the body. This is due to the laxative effect of castor oil. Unfortunately, castor oil does not always succeed in excreting the entire bile completely. The enterohepatic circulation circulates through the body 5-10 times a day and one can imagine that even with castor oil it would be difficult to excrete 100% of the bile. Because that is exactly our goal. Therefore, it is important to combine the castor oil with medicinal charcoal. This causes the released toxins to be bound in the intestine and can therefore no longer be reabsorbed.

How to detox with castor oil: The instruction

You need per session:

1 50ml castor oil

2 50 ml soy milk*

3 Cocoa powder (with emulsifier)

4 a 100 ml medicine bottle with a wide neck (you can get it in any pharmacy). This is reusable and a one-time purchase!

5 Optional: 10 g medicinal charcoal

* If you don't like cocoa and/or soy milk at all, you can use carrot juice instead (then without cocoa powder, of course). I think cow milk instead of soy milk is harmful to health, but it would still be suitable for detoxification. However, I do not recommend it! Cocoa is great for this purpose because the cocoa powder contains emulsifiers that mix with the solid castor oil. In addition, the cocoa masks the unpleasant taste of the castor oil. With carrot juice you don't have this emulsification. So you already feel when swallowing that it is a greasy oil, which can possibly be uncomfortable!

And this is how you proceed:

1. Take the 100 ml medicinal bottle
2. Fill this half (i.e. 50 ml) with soy milk
3. add about 2 teaspoons of cocoa powder
4. close the bottle and shake vigorously
5. now pour in 50ml castor oil
6. shake vigorously again
7. then drink up quickly

When is the best time to take it?

Between 11pm and 2am. You can find out why this time is so important in the chapter "The organ clock". Unfortunately, many people make the mistake of taking castor oil in the morning, around 6 or even 10 a.m. That's very bad. From my own experience I can say that such intake times have such an unfavorable effect that the diarrhea can even extend to the following day! It is therefore better to take the castor oil in the evening before going to bed. And you will see that they will wake up sometime between 6am and 10am in the morning. There will be 1-2 hours of diarrhea, but then the matter is settled and you can go about your day as usual and have no loss of time. If you like, you can do the castor oil detox every week or more often.

A castor oil additive is medicinal charcoal, also known as "activated charcoal". This is carbon, which is in the form of a light, deep black powder that is free of coarse particles. The activated carbon is insoluble in almost all solvents. Medicinal charcoal is obtained from plants through carbonization processes. The charcoal has adsorbing properties, binds various toxins (as well as bacteria) and excretes them in the stool. The

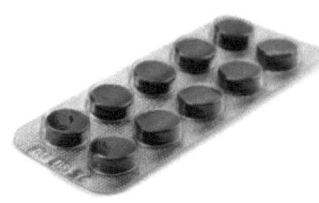

Medicinal charcoal tablets are available cheaply in drugstores

absorption of the toxic bile, which is released into the duodenum by castor oil, is therefore immediately bound so that it can no longer enter the bloodstream. At least that's the theory. The activated charcoal is only effective in the digestive tract and is not absorbed into the blood. Do not take the charcoal tablets at the same time as medication, as they can then become ineffective! The effect of charcoal is controversial. Most reviews of castor oil are based on taking it without medicinal charcoal. Some people believe in an additional detoxification effect, but this has never been confirmed by studies or field reports. The timing of the intake is also controversial and is handled differently by everyone. Some you use 24 hours before, others at the same time as the castor oil. Unfortunately, I cannot give you any advice in this regard, as there are no meaningful empirical values and studies. In any case, the charcoal also has negative effects as it inhibits the absorption of important vitamins and minerals (and medicines). However, this is not a problem if you only take it 1 day a week.

Anyone who deals intensively with castor oil will not be able to avoid the topic of prostaglandins. But why actually? What does castor oil have to do with prostaglandins? And what are prostaglandins anyway? So let's start from the beginning: prostaglandins are tissue hormones that are not produced in a specific organ and then sent into the bloodstream, but are formed in the tissue directly on site. The body needs building materials to produce it. And these are the two essential fatty acids linoleic acid (omega 6) and alpha-linolenic acid (omega 3). But since a picture says more than 1000 words, I have shown the prostaglandin synthesis in the following graphic:

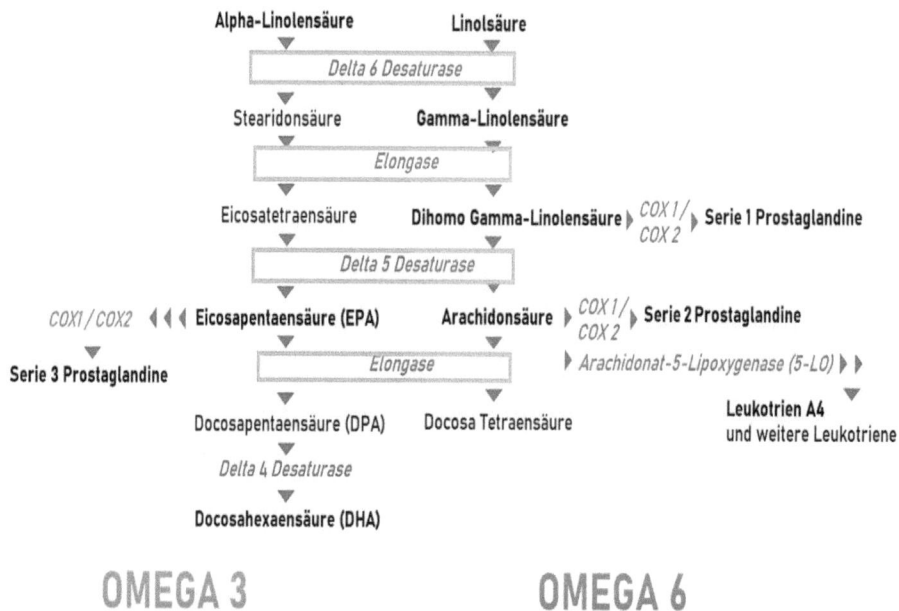

Using enzymes, the starting substance alpha-linolenic acid (omega 3) is transformed into eicosapentaenoic acid (EPA) and from there series 3 prostaglandins. Linoleic acid (omega 6) is further metabolized to arachidonic acid and from there to series 2 prostaglandins The so-called anti-inflammatory series 1 prostaglandins can only be formed using borage oil and/or evening primrose oil. The body always needs the enzymes cyclooxygenase-1 (COX-1) and cyclooxygenase-2 (COX-2) to produce prostaglandins. If these are inhibited (e.g. by aspirin, cetirizine or thyme oil, etc.), only cyclooxygenase-1 is still active. There are also cyclooxygenase inhibitors that inhibit both forms. However, nowadays more selective inhibitors are common, which only inhibit COX-2. That also makes sense, because COX-2 is always formed where inflammation occurs or has already occurred. By inhibiting COX-2, conventional medicine wants to suppress inflammation. Previously there were no selective COX-2 inhibitors in the pharmaceutical industry. Although selective COX2 inhibitors have always existed in nature, such as thyme oil, this has not been of interest to the pharmaceutical industry. The pharmaceutical industry has only been offering selective COX-2 inhibitors for a few years, which do not affect the blocking of COX-1. This is very important because prostaglandins are by no means only involved in inflammation. They have a variety of tasks in the entire organism such as protecting the stomach, blood circulation, bone metabolism and much more. Let's take a closer look at which prostaglandin has which tasks:

Prostaglandin E1: This is the most important prostaglandin for increasing blood flow. It is even used in emergency medicine under the name "alprostadil" to treat acute circulatory disorders. It widens the vessels and, in the event of poor blood circulation, new blood vessels are formed with the help of the VEGF protein (vascular endothelial growth factor). It also inhibits platelet aggregation (the clumping of blood platelets), inhibits proliferation (cell reproduction) and increases it cAMP (cyclic adenosine monophosphate) in many tissues. It also activates the T-lymphocytes (these are the lymphocytes that are formed in the thymus), so prostaglandin E1 also strengthens the immune system and bone metabolism is also stimulated by the E-prostaglandins (study 19). It should also be mentioned that prostaglandin E1 is 20 times stronger than prostaglandin E2 (study P333) and that the ratio of both prostaglandins is usually unfavorably shifted (too much E2, too little E1). So far (as of 2017), it has been disputed whether both prostaglandins bind to the same receptors (EP1, EP2, EP3 and EP4). Due to the current study situation, however, everything points to this (study 333). That means: Both prostaglandins compete for the same receptors!

Prostaglandin E2: ALMOST as good for blood circulation as E1, and in addition, prostaglandin E2 forms a neutralizing mucus that protects the stomach and esophagus (study P20). If you often have heartburn (reflux), then a prostaglandin E2 deficiency could be the cause. In addition, prostaglandin E2 has very regulating properties on the immune system and also causes new blood vessel formation, similar to prostaglandin E1. Various studies have shown that prostaglandin E2 leads to a significant increase in blood flow in the kidneys (study P1) and bone metabolism is also stimulated by E-prostaglandins (study P19).

Prostaglandin D2: Promotes sleep, inhibits platelet aggregation (blood platelets clumping together), promotes vasodilation (widening of blood vessels) in the kidney and bronchoconstriction (narrowing of blood vessels in the bronchi, hence the link with asthma) and promotes water reabsorption in the body small intestine And although it's a type 2 prostaglandin, scientists have found that prostaglandin D2, made from arachidonic acid, has anti-inflammatory effects (Study P30). And the so-called "inflammatory" prostaglandins not only initiate inflammation, but also ensure that it ends again. So you're doing your body a disservice by blocking "inflammatory" prostaglandins like conventional COX inhibitors do.

Prostaglandin I2 (prostacyclin): PGI2, together with PGE2, is the main prostaglandin involved in the inflammatory process. It increases vascular permeability (permeability of blood vessels, which causes tissue swelling), participates in the development of redness and increases pain. Prostacyclin is the strongest platelet aggregation inhibitor and therefore protects against thrombosis like no other prostaglandin! Prostacyclin improves and suppresses blood circulation. It is mainly formed in the vascular endothelium and smooth muscles and has a blood vessel dilating, cell proliferation inhibiting and cell protecting effect.

Prostaglandin F2-alpha: Promotes smooth muscle contraction and is understood as an antagonist to prostaglandin E2.

Thromboxane A2: Can be viewed as the antagonist of prostaglandin I2 (prostacyclin). It is mainly formed by platelets and promotes platelet aggregation. This is important so that you don't bleed to death in the event of injuries (to put it bluntly). It also causes vasoconstriction.

The actual effect only occurs when the prostaglandins dock to the receptors:

After the prostaglandins have been produced, they dock onto receptors ("keyholes") and it is only now that the actual effect occurs.

What role does castor oil play in prostaglandin synthesis?

As you have now learned, the body needs essential fatty acids to produce prostaglandins. That's just 2 (linolenic acid and alpha-linolenic acid). Both are not found in castor oil or only in very small amounts. Nevertheless, castor oil is a real prostaglandin E2 booster. But how does it do that?

1.) Castor oil stimulates the formation of prostaglandin E2 from cell membranes: It encourages the arachidonic acid located in the cell membranes to synthesize prostaglandin E2 from it (study P18a)

2.) Castor oil is half a prostaglandin E2 itself (Study 5):

Substances that have the same pharmaceutical effects as the original are called analogues. Although castor oil with the ricinoleic acid it contains is by no means a prostaglandin, it is at least partly so. Because it independently docks to 2 of the 4 prostaglandin E receptors. Namely on EP3 and EP4 (study 5). The receptors EP1 and EP2 are not occupied by castor oil itself. However, as already described above, castor oil encourages the organism to produce prostaglandin E2 itself. And the original prostaglandin E2 then occupies all 4 receptors. Stimulating the EP3 and EP4 receptors is primarily responsible for hair growth and induction of labor in pregnancy. That is why castor oil is also very popular as a hair restorer and to induce labor during pregnancy (labor cocktail). That's the big secret behind it.

Ill due to prostaglandin deficiency: castor oil as a savior?

You've read all the good reviews about castor oil. Do you really think all of this came about through detoxification? If so, why don't patients who use other detoxification methods also report successes such as curing myopia or increased hair growth? And how should the detoxifying effect actually come about when applied externally? Because castor oil also works externally and this neither interrupts the enterohepatic circulation nor does it detoxify the intestines. It is therefore more likely that castor oil acts due to its prostaglandin E2 booster activity. But can it really be that so many people are deficient in prostaglandins? It is always said that we are supposedly oversupplied with omega-6 fatty acids and that the only thing missing is the so-called anti-inflammatory omega 3. But is that really the case? Let's take a look at which diseases are associated with which prostaglandin deficiencies:

Disease:	Missing prostaglandin:
Poor hair growth, sparse eyebrows and eyelashes	E1, E2, F2-alpha
Glaucoma (increased pressure in the eye)	F2-alpha
Circulatory disorders	E1, E2, I2
Thrombosis	I2
Initiation of childbirth	E2
Grey hair	E2, F2a
Trigeminal neuralgia	E1
Autoimmune diseases	E1, Thromboxan A2
Cancer	E1, A1
Acne	E1
Premenstrual syndrome	E1

Autoimmune diseases also affected by prostaglandin deficiency:

In autoimmune diseases, hyperactivity of B cells (white blood cells made in the bone marrow) and a concomitant loss of regulatory control by T cells (white blood cells made in the thymus) have been found. Prostaglandins are known to regulate the immune response. Deficiencies in prostaglandin E1 and/or thromboxane A2 activate B cells and suppress T cell function. Viruses also play an important role in the pathogenesis of autoimmune diseases. It is known that viruses block the enzyme delta-6-desaturase, which is necessary for prostaglandin E1 synthesis, and thus reduce the cell-mediated immune response (study P10).

As you can see, it is very likely that many diseases are caused by a prostaglandin deficiency. Therefore, it is important to boost prostaglandin synthesis again. Unfortunately, this is not enough with castor oil alone, because castor oil only gives the impulse for prostaglandin production without supplying the building material for it. You need the two essential fatty acids omega 6 and omega 3. However, omega 6 is not the same as omega 6 and omega 3 is not the same as omega 3. Because essential, i.e. vital, are only 2 fatty acids:

• **Alpha Linolenic Acid (Omega 3)**

• **Linoleic acid (Omega 6)**

The body can produce all other fatty acids itself!

This also applies to saturated and monounsaturated fatty acids (omega 9), such as those found in olive oil. Therefore, olive oil has no health benefits. If you now say "yes, but we consume so much omega 6 fatty acids through our modern diet", then I would advise you to take a closer look. Let's start with linoleic acid (omega 6):

- Grapeseed oil approx. 65%

- Safflower oil (safflower oil) approx. 65%

- Hemp oil approx. 50%

- Soybean oil approx. 55%

- Cottonseed oil approx. 50%

- Wheat germ oil approx. 50%

- corn oil approx. 50%

- Sunflower oil approx. 60%

- Sunflower oil for frying about 5%

- rapeseed oil approx. 25%

- Linseed oil approx. 15%

- Olive oil approx. 5%

- walnuts approx. 34%

- Peanuts approx. 14%

- hazelnuts approx. 8%

That means you would have to eat 100g of walnuts a day to get 34g of linoleic acid. Or drink 100 ml of grape seed oil to get 65 g. But I wouldn't recommend it to you, because grapeseed oil is the most contaminated oil with pesticides and unfortunately this also applies to organic oils. The consumer protection magazines reported! With sunflower oil we have a special feature: While the "natural" sunflower oil has a very high linoleic acid content of up to approx. 70%, the sunflower oil used for frying usually has just around 2%-5% (in approximately). Because the linoleic acid is not suitable for frying. That's why they were bred out. So as you can see: it's not that easy to get linoleic acid, as we're told again and again! Linoleic acid is in short supply. And even if you do get enough of it, you may well have an enzyme deficiency that can't further convert linoleic acid to arachidonic acid and prostaglandins. Another way to get series two prostaglandins is to ingest pure arachidonic acid from animal foods, especially lard and offal. But who eats these anyway? Quite apart from all the downsides of the dangerous "meat mafia" with factory farming, growth hormones and antibiotics.

Now let's look at where the second essential fatty acid, omega 3 alpha-linolenic acid, is found:

- Linseed oil: approx. 60%

- Chia oil: approx. 60%

- Perilla oil: approx. 60%

- Sacha Inchi Oil: approx. 50%

- camelina oil: approx. 35%

- Hemp oil: approx. 15%

- Walnut oil: approx. 13%

- Rapeseed oil: approx. 9%

- Soybean oil: approx. 8%

So you can already see that there is a lack of both omega 3 and omega 6. Omega-6 fatty acids are always wrongly presented as "bad" and pro-inflammatory, which is not true per se. It is easy to explain why these two fatty acids are so important: they are involved in the formation of what are known as eicosanoids. These are hormones that are formed locally in the tissue and fulfill a whole range of tasks in the organism. The main tissue hormones are the prostaglandins. However, if there is a lack of linoleic acid (omega 6) and/or alpha-linolenic acid (omega 3), then only insufficient prostaglandins and other eicosanoids are formed. As a result, numerous health problems arise.

Under what criteria are which prostaglandins formed?

- By consuming most of the oils containing linoleic acid (sunflower oil, safflower oil, grapeseed oil), arachidonic acid is always formed and from this the series 2 prostaglandins (and ONLY series 2)! It is not yet clear why this is so. (Study P12)

- If an oil is consumed in which the gamma-linolenic acid is already present (borage oil, evening primrose oil, currant seed oil), series 1 prostaglandins are formed from this (study P16). However, there are no vegetable oils that contain only gamma-linolenic acid alone. Because all oils where gamma-linolenic acid occurs also contain extremely high amounts of linoleic acid, which in turn is converted to arachidonic acid. Oils where gamma-linolenic acid (GLA) is already present are: borage oil (20-25% GLA), black currant seed oil (15-20% GLA) and evening primrose oil (10% GLA).

- If, in addition to the gamma-linolenic acid (borage oil, evening primrose oil...), omega-3 fatty acids are also consumed (namely the already metabolized EPA and DHA from salmon oil), then the gamma-linolenic acid becomes even more (so-called anti-inflammatory) Series 1 prostaglandins formed. In one study, administration of borage oil + salmon oil resulted in 73 nmol/mg of prostaglandin E1, compared to 39.7 nmol/mg when borage oil was administered alone. When given alone, evening primrose oil was only 29 nmol/mg and when corn oil (rich in omega 6 linoleic acid but does not contain gamma linolenic acid such as borage oil) alone, it was less than 0.1 nmol/mg Prostaglandin E1 (study P13).

Why healthy people don't get inflammation from omega 6

After consuming omega-6-rich food, the arachidonic acid accumulates in cell membranes and is converted from there into series 2 prostaglandins (especially prostaglandins I2 and E2) when needed. Two enzymes are required for the conversion of arachidonic acid to prostaglandins:

Cyclooxygenase 1 (COX-1) as well

Cyclooxygenase 2 (COX-2)

The difference between these two enzymes is easily explained: COX-1 is found in tissues throughout the body. COX-2 additionally in inflamed tissue. While prostaglandin E2 synthesis via COX-1 performs more normal, routine activities to maintain bodily functions, such as the formation of neutralizing mucus in the stomach or a blood circulation-promoting effect, only the route via COX-2 promotes inflammation. Therefore, healthy people can consume a lot of omega-6-rich linoleic acid without getting inflammation, while in sick people (e.g. arthrosis, gout, etc.) the linoleic acid can possibly lead to stronger symptoms of the disease. Many people believe that omega 6 is fundamentally at the root of their inflammatory disease. But from my point of view that is definitely not the case. Because healthy people do not feel any inflammation under a high linoleic acid-rich diet. These cannot occur at all because the COX-2 enzyme is missing and this is only synthesized in inflamed tissue. The COX-2 is therefore not formed by the omega-6 linoleic acid, but was already there and was synthesized in the tissue by inflammation (e.g. sunburn). The causes of the inflammation lie elsewhere. Usually in chronic poisoning (or sunburn, for example). When people get pimples after consuming a lot of omega-6-rich vegetable oil, it's usually because of the pesticides they contain or because they've fried the oil. Of course, one shouldn't be surprised if inflammation develops, because polyunsaturated fatty acids are very unstable. They are very susceptible to oxidation. Grape seed oil is said to be particularly heavily contaminated with pesticides. This even applies to BIO oils. The consumer protection institutes reported. In any case, organic oils are preferable to conventional ones.

There are no pro-inflammatory prostaglandins

To this day, there is a widespread misconception that series 1+3 prostaglandins are anti-inflammatory, while series 2 (from arachidonic acid) have a pro-inflammatory effect. But when you read the scientific publications and the numerous testimonials from people who consumed high doses of omega 6, you cannot assume that omega 6 is pro-inflammatory. Rather, prostaglandins have an immunoregulatory effect. In a 2009 study, scientists found that series 2 prostaglandins (particularly prostaglandin D2 and F2-alpha) also have anti-inflammatory effects (Study 30). However, since inflamed tissue is rich in the enzyme cyclooxygenase-2 (COX-2), prostaglandins are increasingly produced in

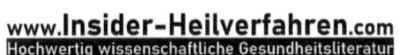

inflamed areas of the body. In any case, one should not think that prostaglandins are the cause of inflammation! Because the inflammation must already have been there before excessive prostaglandin production can take place. COX-2 is also found in other parts of the body (e.g. in the spinal cord, even if there is no inflammation). But for omega 6 to cause inflammation at all, there must have been an inflammation beforehand! And even then, it's not as if omega 6 causes endless inflammation. Rather, a healing is initiated and this is also confirmed by the experience reports. Thus, omega-6 fatty acids can never be the cause of inflammation. This is really far-fetched!

Beware of nonsteroidal anti-inflammatory drugs

I advise against taking so-called COX inhibitors (e.g. aspirin, diclofenac, etc.). It inhibits the enzymes needed for prostaglandin production. And so, taking these drugs leads to a prostaglandin deficiency. The selective COX-2 inhibitors can also lead to serious side effects such as heart attacks or strokes. However, there are natural COX-2 inhibitors from nature such as oregano oil, thyme oil (study 725), lemongrass oil (study 728) or garlic (study 726, 727). These usually have no side effects and even protect against heart attacks and strokes. However, very high doses can (too) thin the blood. Tell your doctor if you are taking high doses of natural COX-2 inhibitors. Essential oils should not be taken more than 5-10 drops per day! Slowly approach how well you tolerate them. Lemongrass oil is the mildest of the remedies listed. While garlic, thyme and oregano oil are very spicy.

If inflammations occur more frequently in the body, then there are completely different reasons (usually too much uric acid and/or toxins, bacteria, viruses, fungi, etc.). But not too much omega 6 or prostaglandins. Inhibiting this is therefore only short-term suppression of symptoms and worsens the health situation even further (study P66a). Nature's COX-2 inhibitors have a different mechanism of action that is not fully understood. Possibly by killing the microbes and relieving the burden on the immune system, among other things.

The enzyme deficiency

A total of 4 different enzymes ensure that the starting substances (linoleic acid / omega 6) or alpha-linolenic acid (omega 3) form the other intermediate metabolic products and finally the arachidonic acid or eicosapentaenoic acid (EPA), from which the prostaglandins are ultimately formed. In other words: If there is already a lack of the 1st enzyme, delta-6 desaturase, no prostaglandins are formed at all! Now, some will probably have fun and think, "That's wonderful. Then I won't need any more aspirin." Unfortunately, it's not that wonderful. The body urgently needs prostaglandins, as I have already explained in detail in this book.

But if the first two enzymes, delta-6 desaturase and elongase, are active and only the 3rd enzyme (delta-5 desaturase) is missing, it wouldn't be that bad. After all, the body could still use it to form series 1 prostaglandins and, if fish oil is consumed, also series 3 prostaglandins. But of course that is not our goal. Because we want all 3 prostaglandin series. So now it's a matter of rebuilding the organism to such an extent that all enzymes function correctly again.

In addition to diabetics, who almost always have these enzyme deficiencies (study P222), it is assumed that people who consume a lot of arachidonic acid through food (i.e. who consume many animal products) also have this enzyme deficiency, since the body presumably thinks that it is no longer needs this enzyme, since enough "ready" arachidonic acid is consumed. These people are anything but prostaglandin 2 deficient. They should have more than enough of that. What is missing in these people are the prostaglandins of series 1. Because these can only be formed using plant-based omega 6 oils, in particular borage oil, evening primrose oil and blackcurrant oil. Ideally together with fish oil. However, with the sole consumption of fish (oil) + arachidonic acid from meat, prostaglandin 1 production does not occur.

And this is how you boost the enzyme activity of the Delta 5 and 6 desaturase back on:

With moderate calorie intake *(increases enzyme activity by 300%)*
Vitamin B3
Vitamin B6
Zinc
Vitamin C
Melatonin (The „sleep hormone")

(Study 222)

Of course, the easiest way to get the nutrients is through a multivitamin supplement. Or you consume foods in which these nutrients are found in increased amounts. On the following pages you will find the nutrient tables.

Vitamin B3 (niacin) comes in two different forms: nicotinic acid and nicotinamide. The former is responsible for the so-called "flush", i.e. the reddening of the skin due to vasodilatation (vasodilatation), triggered by the tissue hormone prostaglandin D2. However, this requires very high doses of at least 100 mg, which can hardly be absorbed through normal nutrition. With the second form, nicotinamide, there is no such flush effect. Niacin is extremely important for the proper functioning of the central nervous system, neuronal development and function. It also regulates cholesterol levels: HDL (so-called "good" cholesterol) increases while pathological cholesterol levels (LDL and triglycerides) are reduced. It reduces the incidence of cardiovascular events, premature aging and age-related neurological disorders such as Alzheimer's, amyotrophic lateral sclerosis, muscle wasting, Parkinson's and malignant glioma (types of brain tumors, glia = supporting tissue of the nervous system). A special feature of vitamin B3 is that it can also be produced by the body itself using the amino acid tryptophan (one of the 8 - 10 essential amino acids). The liver can produce 1 mg of niacin from 60 mg of tryptophan. That means: 600 mg of this amino acid produces 10 mg of niacin, which roughly corresponds to the daily requirement of an adult. Niacin is relatively stable to heat, cooking, and prolonged storage.

Vitamin B3 (niacin) in plant foods:

Rice bran	**34 mg**
Wheat bran flakes	**16 mg**
Roasted Peanuts	**14 mg**
Dried Shiitake Mushrooms	**14 mg**
Peanut butter	**13 mg**
Dried Spirulina Algae	**12 mg**
Paprika	**10 mg**
Hemp seeds	**9 mg**
Sun dried tomatoes	**9 mg**
Chia seeds	**8 mg**
sunflower seeds	**8 mg**
Orange juice	**5 mg**
Pumpkin seeds	**5 mg**
Wheat germ	**5 mg**

All information per 100 g
(Source: US DEPARTMENT OF AGRICULTURE)

Recommended daily intake for adults: **15 mg/day**

Vitamin B6 (pyridoxine) is essential for more than 100 enzymes involved in metabolism. The term vitamin B6 refers to different forms:

- Pyridoxamine
- Pyridoxal
- Pyridoxine

Pyridoxal phosphate (pyridoxal-5'-phosphate / p5P) is the active form of vitamin B6: the liver converts vitamin B6 into the active form P-5-P. For people who have impaired liver function or an enzyme deficiency, it can be helpful to take vitamin B6 as a dietary supplement in the active form as P-5-P. The vitamin is also a coenzyme of numerous enzymatic reactions and important for the regulation of the immune system, for a constant blood sugar level, lipid metabolism, for the formation of the red blood pigment hemoglobin and also plays an important role in lowering the homocysteine level (together with vitamin B4, B9 and B12).

Vitamin B6 (pyridoxine) in plant foods:

Rice bran	4,0 mg
Paprika	2,0 mg
Yeast	2,0 mg
Pistachios	1,7 mg
Bran flakes	1,7 mg
Wheat germ	1,3 mg
Sunflower seeds	1,3 mg
Dried Shiitake Mushrooms	1,0 mg
Sesame	0,8 mg
Dried chestnuts	0,7 mg
Hazelnuts	0,6 mg
Hemp seeds	0,6 mg
Linseed	0,5 mg
Peanuts	0,5 mg
Cashew nuts	0,4 mg

All information per 100 g
(Source: US DEPARTMENT OF AGRICULTURE)

Recommended daily intake for adults: **1.4 - 1.6 mg**

Zinc is a very important trace element for the human body. Zinc deficiency is now known around the world as a malnutrition problem. Bioavailability plays an important role in absorption. The most important inhibitor of zinc absorption is phytic acid (inositol hexaphosphate and pentaphosphate). This is a secondary plant substance that occurs in the outer layers of legumes, cereals and many seeds. Phytic acid is the most important storage form of phosphorus in legumes, grains and nuts. The phytin content can be significantly reduced by soaking in water at 20 degrees for 12 hours. However, only with cereals and legumes, not with nuts! A study (36) did not find a reduced phythin content in nuts, which is why soaking them is not worthwhile. In contrast to phytic acid, proteins increase zinc absorption. The most important deficiency symptoms include anemia (low blood count), hypogonadism (insufficient sex hormones) and dwarfism. Zinc is particularly important for the immune system, for skin, hair and nails, for wound healing, for the formation of hormones such as testosterone and for sperm production.

Zinc in plant foods:

Wheat bran	**13 mg**
Wheat germ	**12 mg**
Yeast	**8mg**
Pumpkin seeds	**7 mg**
Dried chanterelle	**6 mg**
Sunflower seeds	**5 mg**
Cashews	**4 mg**
Porcini dried	**5 mg**
Soybeans	**4 mg**
Oatmeal	**4 mg**
Brazil nuts	**4 mg**
Millet	**3 mg**
Peanuts	**3 mg**
Wheat semolina	**3 mg**
Peanut butter	**3 mg**

All information per 100 g
(Source: US DEPARTMENT OF AGRICULTURE)

Recommended daily intake for adults: **10-16 mg/day**

Vitamin C, also known as ascorbic acid, is a water-soluble vitamin that is essential for development and growth. It also helps repair tissues in the body. For example, the dermal papilla cells are important cells in the skin and hair follicles that provide them with nutrients. The density of these cells continues to decrease over the course of life. Vitamin C is one of the few agents that can condense the density of these dermal papilla cells back to adolescent levels (Study 37). However, the Vit. C must be applied externally, the PH value should be below 3.5 (very acidic) and it must be freshly mixed before application, as it spoils quickly. The thickening of the papilla cells means that it acts against wrinkles and theoretically also allows hair (scalp hair, beard hair, etc.) to grow. Unfortunately, studies and field reports on the subject of hair growth have so far been lacking, so it is not yet certain whether it is effective in this respect. Vitamin C also helps build collagen, strengthens and repairs blood vessel walls. A deficiency is associated with the disease scurvy, which causes brittle blood vessels from which one can bleed and eventually die. But such a massive lack of vitamin C is rare. Moderate chronic deficiencies are much more common. Vitamin C also activates the immune system's killer cells. It acts as a pro-oxidant in high doses and as an antioxidant in moderate amounts, preventing free radical damage. However, this usually only works in combination with secondary plant substances, e.g. in the form of orange juice (which can also be enriched with additional vitamin C!). However, vitamin C taken in isolation has hardly any antioxidant effect and may even have a pro-oxidative effect. In a study on seven subjects, DNA damage was induced using hydrogen peroxide (H_2O_2) and the aim was to find out whether vitamin C in isolation, a sugar drink or a glass of blood orange juice was able to prevent the DNA damage. And at the end of the experiment, it turned out that only the blood orange juice was able to do this (Study 35).

Vitamin C in plant foods:

Australian bush plum	3,000 mg
Camu Camu	2,000 mg
Acerola cherries / juice	1,677 mg
Rosehips	426 mg
Sweet yellow peppers	183 mg
Dried lychees	183 mg
Black Currants	181 mg
Komatsuna	130 mg
Sweet red peppers	127 mg
Oat bran flakes	127 mg
Kiwis	120 mg
Sun dried tomatoes	101 mg
Kale	93 mg
Broccoli	89 mg
Grape juice and orange juice	30 mg

All information per 100 g
(Source: US DEPARTMENT OF AGRICULTURE, etc.)

Recommended daily intake for adults: **1,000 – 5,000 mg/day**

Based on traditional Chinese medicine, the organs receive specific focal points of activity depending on the time:

11 p.m - 1a.m:	**Bile and spleen**
1 - 3 p.m.:	**Liver**
3 - 5 p.m.:	Lungs
5 - 7 p.m.:	Large intestine
7 - 9 p.m.:	Stomach
9 - 11 a.m.:	Pancreas
11am - 1pm:	Heart
1 - 3 p.m.:	Small intestine
3 - 5 p.m.:	Bubble
5 - 7 p.m.:	Kidney
7 - 9 p.m.:	Circuit
9 - 11 p.m.:	Triple heater

The best time to drain with castor oil would therefore be between 11 p.m. and 3 a.m. at night. Unfortunately, many people make the mistake of using castor oil in the morning to laze off. From my own experience, however, I can only strongly advise against it. In such a case, the diarrhea extends to the following day, the diarrhea occurs very suddenly and you may not have a toilet nearby. However, if you drain in accordance with the organ clock, you will have diarrhea for about 30-60 minutes in the morning and that's it. The diarrhea does not extend to the following day, the intestines are completely emptied and you will feel like a new person!

Most people who detox with castor oil do it once a week. Usually at the weekend. But you can also detoxify your body on the other 6 days a week. In addition to castor oil, we have a whole range of other resources available that strengthen and accelerate detoxification with castor oil. You can also use all of these remedies on "castor oil day", i.e. 7 days a week.

Modified citrus pectin

Pectins are gel-forming polysaccharides (multiple sugars) from plant cell walls, especially apple and citrus fruits. Pectins are a type of dietary fiber and vary in the length of their polysaccharide chains, from 300-1000 monosaccharides. Because pectins are not digestible by humans, the modified citrus pectin is chemically altered (hence the name "modified") to increase absorbency. The pectin is changed by increasing the PH value and increasing the temperature. The resulting smaller molecule consists predominantly of D-polygalacturonate and is more easily absorbed by the human digestive system. Most people use pectin as a gelling agent in fruit preserves and jellies. In fact, many of the chemical properties that pectin finds in cooking are similar to those found in modified citrus pectin. It is a chemically modified form of pectin that is particularly rich in sugar molecules known as galactosides. Galectin-3 molecules interact specifically with those galactosides found in modified citrus pectin. In this way, pectin acts as an inhibitor of galectin-3, thus preventing the actions that can damage your health. The intestine cannot absorb pectin in its natural form. This makes it an effective source of fiber. The pectin from citrus fruits is processed to make the molecules smaller so they can more easily enter the bloodstream.

After just one week, 500% increased heavy metal excretion via the urine: There are a number of studies that have demonstrated the effect of modified citrus pectin on removing heavy metals (lead, cadmium and arsenic). A 2008 study concluded that modified citrus pectin is an effective chelator of lead in children hospitalized with toxic levels of lead. Children with a blood serum level of more than 20 mcg/dl received 15 g mod. Citrus pectin (company "PectaSol") in three divided doses per day. There was a dramatic 161% decrease in blood serum lead levels and a dramatic increase in 24-hour urinary excretion (Study 1). In summary, five case studies from 2007 showed a significant reduction in toxic heavy metals (74% average decrease) without any side effects (Study 2). Significant Heavy Metal Excretions Even in Healthy People: Another study was conducted to evaluate the effect of modified citrus pectin on urinary excretion of toxic elements in healthy individuals. The study subjects were daily 15 grams mod. Citrus pectin administered for 5 days. 24-hour urine samples were collected on day 1 and day 6 for comparison to baseline. In the first 24 hours of the mod. Citrus pectin administration significantly increased urinary excretion of arsenic by 130%. On day 6 there was a 150% increase in cadmium excretion. In the case of lead, there was even a 560% increase in excretion in the urine. The remarkable thing about this study was that it was not about sick people with acute metal poisoning, but about normal, healthy subjects! So you can already see that even in supposedly healthy people, heavy metals are hidden, which were only detected and excreted by the modified citrus pectin (study 3). According to studies, modified citrus pectin also works against cancer and metastases. You can find detailed information on the subject of cancer in my book „Insider Cures Against Cancer".

Effect:	Eliminates heavy metals, especially lead, cadmium and arsenic
Recommended dosage:	5 grams 3 times a day for at least 1 month.
Costs:	approx. **50 € / month** if 15 g are consumed per day and one kg is bought for approx. 100 €
Sources of supply:	Health shops
Studies:	(1) (2) (3)

Information provided without guarantee. Use at your own risk!

Tested positive for:

In vitro (test tube)	In vivo (animals)	In vivo (human)
		✔

Garlic

Garlic (Allium sativum) is one of the oldest cultivated plants in the world and has been used medicinally for thousands of years. Many people despise it because of its smell. But its effects on health are gigantic: it has an antimicrobial, antithrombotic, antiarthritic, hypoglycaemic (blood sugar lowering) effect and much more. Garlic is native to Central Asia and northeastern Iran. In the meantime, however, garlic is even cultivated in Germany. The largest garlic producer in the world is China with 79%. The component responsible for the typical garlic smell is the allicin contained in garlic. This smell, which many people dislike, can be prevented or at least mitigated with the help of fresh parsley, sage, cardamom or mint. Garlic isn't all sulfur, as many might think. It contains a whole bunch of nutrients. The adenosine found in garlic is particularly noteworthy. It is a component of ATP (adenosine triphosphate) and as such is important for cell energy production. Adenosine also opens potassium channels, which relax blood vessels, reducing muscle tone and lowering blood pressure. Garlic also stimulates the immune system's T-cells and natural killer cells, thereby strengthening the body's defenses, particularly against cancer and virus-infected cells. Few people know that garlic is also a good antidote to heavy metals (especially lead and cadmium). Treating mice exposed to lead and cadmium with garlic (12.5-100 mg/L) significantly reduced lead and cadmium concentrations in the animals' liver, kidney, heart, spleen and blood organs (Study 11). Furthermore, garlic also activates detoxification enzymes (Study 12).

Effect:	Eliminates heavy metals (especially cadmium and lead) and activates detoxification enzymes. It also has numerous other health-promoting effects such as lowering blood pressure and blood sugar (diabetes) or strengthening the immune system.
Recommended dosage:	At least one tuber every day.
Costs:	If a tuber is eaten every day, count on it about **8 € per month.**
Sources of supply:	In every supermarket
What to look out for:	The garlic smell, which many people dislike, can be prevented or at least mitigated with the help of fresh parsley, sage, cardamom or mint. Be sure to grind the garlic or chew it well, as the active ingredients only become effective when you grind it!
Studies:	**(11) (12)**

Information provided without guarantee. Use at your own risk!

Tested positive for:

In vitro (test tube)	In vivo (animals)	In vivo (human)
	✔	

(R+)-alpha lipoic acid

This is a sulphur-containing fatty acid that has a very strong antioxidant effect (both fat- and water-soluble), which is produced by the body itself. It is involved in numerous enzymes, including sugar and fat metabolism, and is one of the strongest (endogenous) antioxidants. In most cases, however, the amounts produced by the body itself are not sufficient to meet the need (especially in the case of poisoning), so that additional intake through food or in the form of tablets is helpful. The best documented effect is the removal of excess iron from the body. There are also people with an iron deficiency, which can lead to hair loss and anemia, for example. The reverse is also true, namely that there is too much iron in the body. This is very problematic because iron is very reactive. The more iron there is in the body, the higher the oxidative stress from free radicals. Women before menopause (menopause) lose a lot of iron through their menstrual periods, which is very good for their health, while children, men and women after menopause do not have this protection and therefore there is a risk of excess iron. A study (13) showed that women after the menopause had significantly higher iron levels (ferritin) in their skin than in women before the menopause, and the excessively high iron levels correlated with oxidative stress, which damaged cells and also wrinkled skin skin can lead to. Alpha lipoic acid has been found to be effective here (Study 14) because it chemically reacts with iron and wicks it out of the body. The body only needs iron in very small concentrations! Do not take any dietary supplement that contains iron! Unless you have actually been diagnosed with iron deficiency. In addition to alpha-lipoic acid, blood donations and artemisinin are other measures to remove iron from the body. You can find the alpha-lipoic acid in foods such as: spinach, broccoli, rice bran, Brussels sprouts and tomatoes, potatoes and peas.

Effect:	A very strong antioxidant that also wicks excess iron out of the body.
Recommended dosage:	**600 mg daily**, in the morning on an empty stomach
Costs:	about **27 €** / month
Sources of supply:	Health shops and Pharmacies
What to look out for:	Make absolutely sure that it is the (R+) variant trades! Only this is the original. Other forms are synthetically produced and have a much weaker effect! In addition, you should only take the tablets 2 hours after eating or 30 minutes before eating, as food reduces the absorption of alpha-lipoic acid! However, the best thing is to take it in the morning on an empty stomach!
Studies:	**(13) (14) (15) (16)**

Information provided without guarantee. Use at your own risk!

Tested positive for:

In vitro (test tube)	In vivo (animals)	In vivo (human)
		✔

Selenium

Selenium is a vital trace element that we absolutely have to ingest with food because the body cannot produce it itself. Many regions of the world, including Europe, are considered selenium deficiency areas. Large parts of the population are undersupplied with selenium. But an overdose also poses major health risks. Both too much and too little selenium is massively harmful to health, which is why care should be taken to ensure an exact dosage. Selenium is one of the strongest endogenous antioxidants, so it protects cells from oxidative stress and is also involved in numerous enzymes. Above all on glutathione peroxidase, which renders free oxygen radicals harmless. The trace element is suitable both for protecting the cells from heavy metals and for removing them, as was shown in a study (18): The residents of Wanshan, China, suffer from increased mercury levels. The aim of a study was to investigate the effects of oral supplementation with selenium-enriched yeast in this long-term mercury-exposed population. 103 volunteers from the region were recruited and 53 of them were treated with 100 micrograms of organic selenium (as selenium yeast) daily for 3 months, while 50 of them were treated with yeast without selenium. There was a significant increase in the mercury concentrations in the urine in the subjects treated with selenium from the 30th day of treatment, which increased significantly up to the 90th day of treatment. There was no increased excretion of mercury in the groups treated with placebo. And: the greater the burden of heavy metals in the body, the more the selenium level plummets (Study 17). Brazil nuts are particularly rich in selenium with approx. 1,900 micrograms per 100 g.

Selenium in plant foods:

Brazil nuts	**1,917mcg**
Ground mustard seeds	**208 mcg**
Sunflower seeds	**79 mcg**
Wheat germ	**65 mcg**
Chia seeds	**55 mcg**
Whole grain bread	**52 mcg**
Bran flakes	**52 mcg**
Dried Shiitake Mushrooms	**46 mcg**
Oat bran	**45 mcg**
Wholemeal Flatbread	**44 mcg**
Peanut butter	**40 mcg**
Yellow Mustard	**33 mcg**
Oat bran flakes	**26 mcg**
Chocolate drink powder	**21 mcg**
Wheat cream	**20 mcg**

All information per 100 g
(Source: US DEPARTMENT OF AGRICULTURE)

Recommended daily intake for adults: **200 mcg/day**

Effect:	Eliminates mercury and protects cells from heavy metals
Recommended dosage:	**100-200 mcg/day** as selenium yeast. Do not use more, as selenium is toxic in higher doses!
Costs:	2 – 3 € / month
Sources of supply:	Pharmacies and health shops
What to look out for:	Selenium should not be overdosed, otherwise it can have a toxic effect! This also applies to the consumption of food.
Studies:	**(17) (18)**

Information provided without guarantee. Use at your own risk!

Tested positive for:

In vitro (test tube)	In vivo (animals)	In vivo (human)
		✔

Vitamin C

Rats were given a diet with a daily dose of 10 mg cadmium/kg in the diet for 28 days. One group received normal drinking water, the other group drinking water enriched with vitamin C. In the vitamin C group, the cadmium content in the liver, kidneys, testicles and muscles decreased. The highest decreases were found in the testes, the lowest in the muscles (Study 406). Furthermore, vitamin C is also an essential vitamin in other respects, which, for example, strengthens the immune system, keeps blood vessels elastic or promotes collagen formation.

Vitamin C in plant foods:

Australian bush plum	**3,000 mg**
Camu Camu	**2,000 mg**
Acerola cherries / juice	**1,677 mg**
Rosehips	**426 mg**
Sweet yellow peppers	**183 mg**
Dried lychees	**183 mg**
Black Currants	**181 mg**
Komatsuna	**130 mg**
Sweet red peppers	**127 mg**
Oat bran flakes	**127 mg**
Kiwis	**120 mg**
Sun dried tomatoes	**101 mg**
Kale	**93 mg**
Broccoli	**89 mg**
Grape juice and orange juice	**30 mg**

All information per 100 g
(Source: US DEPARTMENT OF AGRICULTURE, etc.)

Recommended daily intake for adults: **1,000 – 5,000 mg/day**

Vitamin C **At a glance ▼**	
Recommended dosage:	**1 – 5 g / day**
Costs:	1 € / month
Sources of supply:	Health shops, Pharmacies
Studies:	(406)

Information provided without guarantee. Use at your own risk!

Tested positive for:

In vitro (test tube)	In vivo (animals)	In vivo (human)
	✔	

Other detoxification options

In particular, chlorella algae, spirulina algae, wild garlic and coriander are very popular in alternative medicine circles and are recommended by many therapists. Unfortunately, I am not aware of any meaningful studies on humans (not even on animals) for these therapies, so I cannot recommend them at this point in time. If you know of a meaningful study, please let me know:

mail@insider-heilverfahren.com

I'll be sure to save this for the next edition!

Overview of the verified scientific findings of the individual agents against heavy metals:					
	Lead	Cadmium	Iron	Arsenic	Mercury
Selenium					✔
Alpha-lipoic acid			✔		
Modified citrus pectin	✔	✔		✔	
Garlic	✔	✔			
Modified citrus pectin + Selenium + Alpha-lipoic acid	✔	✔	✔	✔	✔

(1) The role of modified citrus pectin as an effective chelator of lead in children hospitalized with toxic lead levels.

https://www.ncbi.nlm.nih.gov/pubmed/18616067

(2) Integrative medicine and the role of modified citrus pectin/alginates in heavy metal chelation and detoxification - five case reports.

https://www.ncbi.nlm.nih.gov/pubmed/18219211

(3) The effect of modified citrus pectin on the urinary excretion of toxic elements.

https://www.ncbi.nlm.nih.gov/pubmed/16835878

(4) The mechanism and attenuation of niacin-induced flushing

https://www.ncbi.nlm.nih.gov/pmc/articles/PMC2779993

(5) Castor oil induces laxation and uterus contraction via ricinoleic acid activating prostaglandin EP3 receptors

https://www.ncbi.nlm.nih.gov/pmc/articles/PMC3384204/

(6) Cadmium overload and toxicity

https://www.ncbi.nlm.nih.gov/pubmed/11904357

(7) Cadmium and cancer

https://www.ncbi.nlm.nih.gov/pubmed/23430782

(8) *Toxicity of lead: A review with recent updates*

https://www.ncbi.nlm.nih.gov/pmc/articles/PMC3485653/

(9) *Lead Contamination in Cocoa and Cocoa Products: Isotopic Evidence of Global Contamination*

https://www.ncbi.nlm.nih.gov/pmc/articles/PMC1281277/

(10) *The role of prostaglandin E2-EP3/EP4 receptor signaling in enhancing lymphangiogenesis*

https://pubmed.ncbi.nlm.nih.gov/21311040/

(11) *Garlic (Allium sativum L.) as a potential antidote to cadmium and lead poisoning: distribution and analysis of cadmium and lead in different mouse organs*

https://pubmed.ncbi.nlm.nih.gov/17916975/

(12) *Garlic-derived sodium 2-propenylthiosulfate induces phase II detoxification enzymes in rat hepatoma H4IIE cells*

https://pubmed.ncbi.nlm.nih.gov/20650352/

(13) *Menopause increases the iron storage protein ferritin in the skin*

http://europepmc.org/article/med/23752032

(14) *Alpha-lipoic acid reduces iron-induced toxicity and oxidative stress in an iron overload model*

https://pubmed.ncbi.nlm.nih.gov/30708965/

(15) Oxidative stress and antioxidant therapy with alpha-lipoic acid entrapment in acute 2,4-dichlorophenoxyacetic acid-based herbicide poisoning

https://pubmed.ncbi.nlm.nih.gov/24908976/

(16) Protective function of DL-alpha-lipoic acid against mercury-induced neuronal lipid peroxidation

https://pubmed.ncbi.nlm.nih.gov/10051379/

(17) Relationship between selenium, lead and mercury in red blood cells of Saudi autistic children

https://link.springer.com/article/10.1007/s11011-017-9996-1

(18) Organic selenium supplementation increases mercury excretion and reduces oxidative damage in residents with long-term exposure to mercury from Wanshan, China

https://www.semanticscholar.org/paper/Organic-selenium-supplementation-increases-mercury-Li-Dong/80674a6e70e01d9445ba6a1ee9bae68a94486bb9

(35) Orange juice versus vitamin C: effect on hydrogen peroxide-induced DNA damage in blood mononuclear cells

https://pubmed.ncbi.nlm.nih.gov/17349075/

(406) Effect of vitamin C on cadmium absorption and distribution in rats.

https://www.ncbi.nlm.nih.gov/pubmed/15646266

(725) Carvacrol, a component of thyme oil, activates PPARalpha and gamma and suppresses COX-2 expression

https://pubmed.ncbi.nlm.nih.gov/19578162/

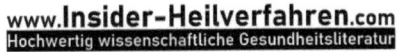

(726) *Aged garlic extract attenuates brain damage and cyclooxygenase-2 induction after ischemia and reperfusion in rats*

https://pubmed.ncbi.nlm.nih.gov/21850441/

(727) *Mechanism by which garlic (Allium sativum) inhibits cyclooxygenase activity. Effect of raw versus cooked garlic extract on the synthesis of prostanoids*

https://pubmed.ncbi.nlm.nih.gov/8821119/

(728) *Citral, a component of lemongrass oil, activates PPARα and γ and suppresses COX-2 expression*

https://pubmed.ncbi.nlm.nih.gov/20656057/

(P1) *Prostaglandin E2 induced changes in renal blood flow, renal interstitial hydrostatic pressure and sodium excretion in the rat.*

https://www.ncbi.nlm.nih.gov/pubmed/2093936

(P10) *Autoimmunity and prostaglandins*

https://www.ncbi.nlm.nih.gov/pubmed/7035343

(P12) *The effects of evening primrose oil, safflower oil and paraffin on plasma fatty acids in humans: choosing an appropriate placebo for clinical trials of primrose oil.*

https://www.ncbi.nlm.nih.gov/pubmed/1871175

(P13) *Mouse peritoneal macrophage prostaglandin E1 synthesis is altered by dietary gamma-linolenic acid.*

https://www.ncbi.nlm.nih.gov/pubmed/1322453

(P16) *Importance of dietary gamma-linolenic acid in human health and nutrition.*

https://www.ncbi.nlm.nih.gov/pubmed/9732298

(P18a) Effect of castor oil diet on prostaglandin E2 synthesis in pregnant rats

https://www.ncbi.nlm.nih.gov/pubmed/11263183

(P19) Prostaglandin E stimulates bone formation

https://www.ncbi.nlm.nih.gov/pmc/articles/PMC2266676/

(P20) Prostaglandin EP receptors and their roles in mucosal protection and ulcer healing in the gastrointestinal tract.

https://www.ncbi.nlm.nih.gov/pubmed/20857620

(P30) The anti-inflammatory effects of prostaglandins

https://www.ncbi.nlm.nih.gov/pubmed/19240648

(P66a) Chronic administration of selective cyclooxygenase-2 (COX-2) inhibitors results in an increased risk of adverse cardiovascular events, including myocardial infarction and stroke

https://www.ncbi.nlm.nih.gov/pubmed/26543101

(P222) Loss of delta-6 desaturase activity as a key factor in aging.

https://www.ncbi.nlm.nih.gov/pubmed/6270521

(P333) Multiple roles of dihomo-?-linolenic acid against proliferative diseases

https://www.ncbi.nlm.nih.gov/pmc/articles/PMC3295719/

2 field reports: Chronic diarrhea and other gastrointestinal complaints

(1a) http://www.symptome.ch/vbboard/entgiftung-allgemein/1804-ricinusoel-6.html

(1b) http://www.symptome.ch/vbboard/entgiftung-allgemein/1804-ricinusoel-179.html

1 field report: eczema

(2a) http://www.symptome.ch/vbboard/entgiftung-allgemein/1804-ricinusoel-26.html

3 testimonials: tinnitus

(3a) http://www.symptome.ch/vbboard/entgiftung-allgemein/1804-ricinusoel-28.html

(3b) http://www.symptome.ch/vbboard/entgiftung-allgemein/1804-ricinusoel-124.html

(3c) http://www.symptome.ch/vbboard/entgiftung-allgemein/1804-ricinusoel-410.html

2 reviews: allergies

(4a) http://www.symptome.ch/vbboard/entgiftung-allgemein/1804-ricinusoel-28.html

(4b) http://www.symptome.ch/vbboard/entgiftung-allgemein/1804-ricinusoel-620.html

2 testimonials: Rosy, firm skin

(5a) http://www.symptome.ch/vbboard/entgiftung-allgemein/1804-ricinusoel-90.html

(5b) http://www.symptome.ch/vbboard/entgiftung-allgemein/1804-ricinusoel-130.html

(5c) http://www.symptome.ch/vbboard/entgiftung-allgemein/1804-ricinusoel-644.html

4 reviews: hair loss and baldness

(6a) http://www.symptome.ch/vbboard/entgiftung-allgemein/1804-ricinusoel-90.html

(6b) http://www.symptome.ch/vbboard/entgiftung-allgemein/1804-ricinusoel-125.html

(6c) http://www.symptome.ch/vbboard/entgiftung-allgemein/1804-ricinusoel-593.html

(6d) http://www.symptome.ch/vbboard/entgiftung-allgemein/1804-ricinusoel-594.html

5 reviews: Acne and impure skin

(7a) http://www.symptome.ch/vbboard/entgiftung-allgemein/1804-ricinusoel-130.html

(7b) http://www.symptome.ch/vbboard/entgiftung-allgemein/1804-ricinusoel-148.html

(7c) http://www.symptome.ch/vbboard/entgiftung-allgemein/1804-ricinusoel-197.html

(7d) http://www.symptome.ch/vbboard/entgiftung-allgemein/1804-ricinusoel-304.html

(7e) http://www.symptome.ch/vbboard/entgiftung-allgemein/1804-ricinusoel-410.html

2 field reports: short-sightedness (myopia)

(8a) http://www.symptome.ch/vbboard/entgiftung-allgemein/1804-ricinusoel-148.html

(8b) http://www.symptome.ch/vbboard/entgiftung-allgemein/1804-ricinusoel-148.html

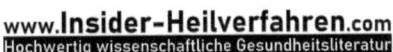

4 testimonials: Chronic fatigue

(9a) http://www.symptome.ch/vbboard/entgiftung-allgemein/1804-ricinusoel-179.html

(9b) http://www.symptome.ch/vbboard/entgiftung-allgemein/1804-ricinusoel-295.html

(9c) http://www.symptome.ch/vbboard/entgiftung-allgemein/1804-ricinusoel-359.html

(9d) http://www.symptome.ch/vbboard/entgiftung-allgemein/1804-ricinusoel-425.html

1 field report: back pain

(10a) http://www.symptome.ch/vbboard/entgiftung-allgemein/1804-ricinusoel-179.html

2 reviews: histamine intolerance

(11a) http://www.symptome.ch/vbboard/entgiftung-allgemein/1804-ricinusoel-253.html

(11b) http://www.symptome.ch/vbboard/entgiftung-allgemein/1804-ricinusoel-295.html

1 field report: Electrosensitivity

(12a) http://www.symptome.ch/vbboard/entgiftung-allgemein/1804-ricinusoel-266.html

1 field report: Extreme sweating

(13a) http://www.symptome.ch/vbboard/entgiftung-allgemein/1804-ricinusoel-295.html

1 experience report: pain in the musculoskeletal system

(14a) http://www.symptome.ch/vbboard/entgiftung-allgemein/1804-ricinusoel-295.html

4 field report: migraine/headache

(15a) http://www.symptome.ch/vbboard/entgiftung-allgemein/1804-ricinusoel-295.html

(15b) http://www.symptome.ch/vbboard/entgiftung-allgemein/1804-ricinusoel-304.html

(15c) http://www.symptome.ch/vbboard/entgiftung-allgemein/1804-ricinusoel-410.html

(15d) http://www.symptome.ch/vbboard/entgiftung-allgemein/1804-ricinusoel-432.html

1 field report: Various intolerances

(16a) http://www.symptome.ch/vbboard/entgiftung-allgemein/1804-ricinusoel-302.html

1 experience report: colds

(17a) http://www.symptome.ch/vbboard/entgiftung-allgemein/1804-ricinusoel-304.html

1 field report: Elevated cadmium levels

(18a) http://www.symptome.ch/vbboard/entgiftung-allgemein/1804-ricinusoel-327.html

1 field report: sleep disorders

(19a) http://www.symptome.ch/vbboard/entgiftung-allgemein/1804-ricinusoel-406.html

1 experience report: pulling in the ear

(20a) http://www.symptome.ch/vbboard/entgiftung-allgemein/1804-ricinusoel-417.html

1 experience report: numbness after heavy work

(21a) http://www.symptome.ch/vbboard/entgiftung-allgemein/1804-ricinusoel-530.html

1 field report: psoriasis (psoriasis)

(22a) http://www.symptome.ch/vbboard/entgiftung-allgemein/1804-ricinusoel-620.html

Photo credits

Cover image oil: © naypong, Fotolia

For all other photos in this book and the cover:

Images licensed by Ingram Image

Imprint

Publisher:
Books on demand / Norderstedt (Germany)

Author and editor:
Christian Meyer-Esch
Insider-Heilverfahren.com,
e-Mail: mail@insider-heilverfahren.com

About the author
Christian Meyer-Esch has been intensively involved with alternative and holistic medicine for 18 years.
He searches for scientific studies and field reports worldwide to find solutions, especially for diseases that are difficult to treat. His main focus is on investigating the causes.

Copyright © 2022
Christian Meyer-Esch

If you have any questions or suggestions, please send me an email:

mail@insider-heilverfahren.com

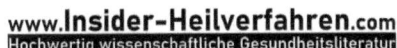

There is space for your documentation here! You always have an exact overview of the number of detoxification sessions that have already been completed. You can enter up to 362 derivations. In the comment field you can enter what health improvements have occurred.

Number:	Date:	Comment:
1.		
2.		
3.		
4.		
5.		
6.		
7.		
8.		
9.		
10.		
11.		
12.		
13.		
14.		
15.		
16.		
17.		
18.		

19.		
20.		
21.		
22.		
23.		
24.		
25.		
26.		
27.		
28.		
29.		
30.		
31.		
32.		
33.		
34.		
35.		
36.		
37.		
38.		
39.		
40.		
41.		
42.		
43.		

44.		
45.		
46.		
47.		
48.		
49.		
50.		
51.		
52.		
53.		
54.		
55.		
56.		
57.		
58.		
59.		
60.		
61.		
62.		
63.		
64.		
65.		
66.		
67.		
68.		

69.		
70.		
71.		
72.		
73.		
74.		
75.		
76.		
77.		
78.		
79.		
80.		
81.		
82.		
83.		
84.		
85.		
86.		
87.		
88.		
89.		
90.		
91.		
92.		
93.		

94.		
95.		
96.		
97.		
98.		
99.		
100.		
101.		
102.		
103.		
104.		
105.		
106.		
107.		
108.		
109.		
110.		
111.		
112.		
113.		
114.		
115.		
116.		
117.		
118.		

119.		
120.		
121.		
122.		
123.		
124.		
125.		
126.		
127.		
128.		
129.		
130.		
131.		
132.		
133.		
134.		
135.		
136.		
137.		
138.		
139.		
140.		
141.		
142.		
143.		

144.		
145.		
146.		
147.		
148.		
149.		
150.		
151.		
152.		
153.		
154.		
155.		
156.		
157.		
158.		
159.		
160.		
161.		
162.		
163.		
164.		
165.		
166.		
167.		
168.		

Healing and Detoxification with Castor Oil

169.		
170.		
171.		
172.		
173.		
174.		
175.		
176.		
177.		
178.		
179.		
180.		
181.		
182.		
183.		
184.		
185.		
186.		
187.		
188.		
189.		
190.		
191.		
192.		
193.		

194.		
195.		
196.		
197.		
198.		
199.		
200.		
201.		
202.		
203.		
204.		
205.		
206.		
207.		
208.		
209.		
210.		
211.		
212.		
213.		
214.		
215.		
216.		
217.		
218.		

219.		
220.		
221.		
222.		
223.		
224.		
225.		
226.		
227.		
228.		
229.		
230.		
231.		
232.		
233.		
234.		
235.		
236.		
237.		
238.		
239.		
240.		
241.		
242.		
243.		

244.		
245.		
246.		
247.		
248.		
249.		
250.		
251.		
252.		
253.		
254.		
255.		
256.		
257.		
258.		
259.		
260.		
261.		
262.		
263.		
264.		
265.		
266.		
267.		
268.		

269.		
270.		
271.		
272.		
273.		
274.		
275.		
276.		
277.		
278.		
279.		
280.		
281.		
282.		
283.		
284.		
285.		
286.		
287.		
288.		
289.		
290.		
291.		
292.		
293.		

294.		
295.		
296.		
297.		
298.		
299.		
300.		
301.		
302.		
303.		
304.		
305.		
306.		
307.		
308.		
309.		
310.		
311.		
312.		
313.		
314.		
315.		
316.		
317.		
318.		

319.		
320.		
321.		
322.		
323.		
324.		
325.		
326.		
327.		
328.		
329.		
330.		
331.		
332.		
333.		
334.		
335.		
336.		
337.		
338.		
339.		
340.		
341.		
342.		
343.		

344.		
345.		
346.		
347.		
348.		
349.		
350.		
351.		
352.		
353.		
354.		
355.		
356.		
357.		
358.		
359.		
360.		
361.		
362.		